NOURISHING START

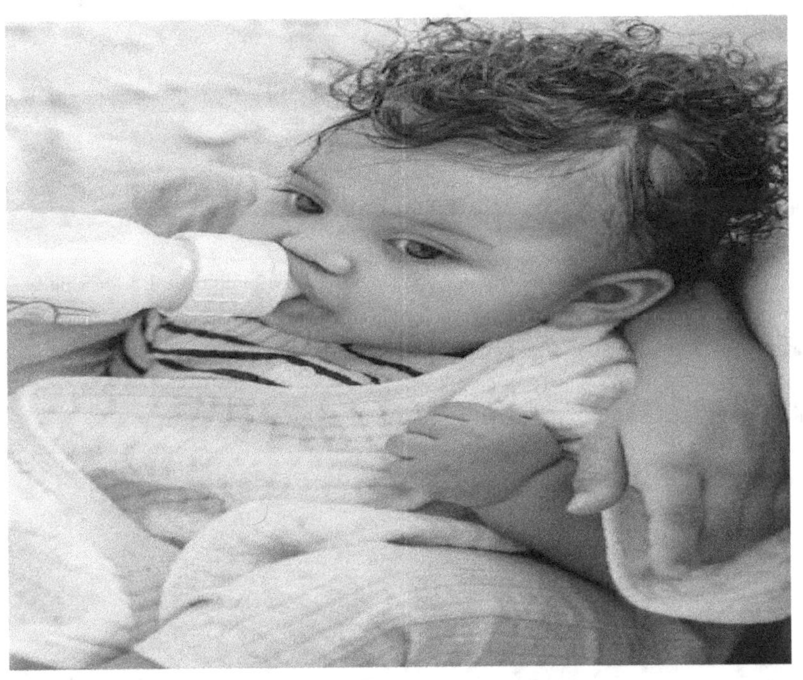

Easy and Tasty Baby
Food ideas for new Mother

Dora Oliver

TABLE OF CONTENT

INTRODUCTION

Welcome to the Culinary Journey of Motherhood

Being a mother is an amazing and life-changing experience filled with many happy and loving moments, as well as the constant need to provide your child with the best. One significant aspect of this journey is navigating the world of baby food and understanding how to nourish your child in the most wholesome and delightful way.

The Significance of Culinary Choices

The culinary journey of motherhood begins with a recognition of the vital role that nutrition plays in a child's early development. Every bite contributes to their growth, cognitive function, and overall well-bei

Embracing Nutrient-Packed Choices

As a new mother, you will discover the joy of crafting meals that not only satisfy your baby's taste buds but also provide essential nutrients for their growth. This journey involves exploring a variety of flavors, textures, and nutrient combinations.

Tailoring Meals to Your Little One

One of the initial steps is to understand the unique needs of your baby. Whether transitioning from breastfeeding to introducing solids, each milestone requires thoughtful consideration of age-appropriate foods and textures.

Building a Foundation of Healthy Habits

The culinary journey of motherhood is an opportunity to instill lifelong healthy eating habits. By introducing a diverse range of fruits, vegetables, and proteins early on, you lay the foundation for a balanced and nutritious diet.

Culinary Creativity for Tiny Taste Buds

Embrace the joy of culinary creativity by experimenting with wholesome purees, finger foods, and engaging meals. This not only nourishes your baby but also turns mealtime into a delightful and interactive experience.

Balancing Nutrition for Both Mother and Child

Beyond the baby's meals, the culinary journey of motherhood extends to maintaining a balanced diet for yourself. Ensuring that you receive the necessary nutrients supports your well-being and, in turn, your ability to care for your little one.

Overcoming Challenges with Knowledge

The journey may present challenges, from picky eaters to concerns about allergies. However, armed with knowledge about age-appropriate foods, allergen introduction, and troubleshooting tips, you can navigate these challenges with confidence.

Celebrating Milestones Through Food

Every spoonful represents a milestone in your baby's development. Whether it's the first taste of solid food or the transition to self-feeding, each moment is an opportunity to celebrate growth and progression.

Importance of Nutritious Baby Food

The significance of providing nutritious baby food cannot be overstated, as it plays a pivotal role in the early stages of a child's development. The choices made during this critical period have far-reaching effects on their growth, health, and future well-being.

Foundation for Growth and Development

Nutritious baby food serves as the foundation for optimal growth and development. Essential nutrients such as vitamins, minerals, and proteins are crucial for the formation of organs, bones, and a robust immune system.

Cognitive Development and Brain Health

The early years are a period of rapid brain development. Nutrient-rich foods, especially those containing omega-3 fatty acids, iron, and zinc, contribute to cognitive function, memory, and overall brain health.

Building Strong Immunity

A well-balanced diet strengthens a baby's immune system, helping them ward off infections and illnesses. Vitamins like A, C, and D, along with minerals like zinc, play a key role in supporting a robust immune response.

Establishing Healthy Eating Habits

Introducing nutritious foods during infancy lays the groundwork for establishing healthy eating habits later in life. Early exposure to a variety of flavors and textures enhances a child's palate and encourages a diverse and balanced diet.

Energy for Active Exploration

Babies are natural explorers, and proper nutrition provides the energy they need for physical activities, motor skill development, and the exploration of their surroundings.

Support for Digestive Health

Nutrient-rich baby foods, including fiber-rich fruits and vegetables, contribute to healthy digestion. This helps prevent constipation and establishes a foundation for good digestive health.

Prevention of Nutritional Deficiencies

Meeting the nutritional needs of a growing baby helps prevent deficiencies that could lead to developmental delays or health issues. Adequate intake of iron, calcium, and other essential nutrients is crucial during this stage.

Role in Allergen Introduction

The introduction of allergenic foods at the right time and in the right way can reduce the risk of allergies. Nutritious baby food includes a gradual introduction to potential allergens, promoting tolerance and minimizing the likelihood of allergic reactions.

Emotional Connection and Bonding

The act of providing nutritious meals fosters a strong emotional connection between the caregiver and the baby. Shared mealtime experiences create a positive association with food and reinforce the bond between parent and child.

Setting the Stage for a Healthy Future

Nutritious baby food is not just about meeting immediate needs; it's an investment in the child's long-term health and well-being. Healthy eating habits established in infancy contribute to a foundation for a healthy future.

CHAPTER 1

Kitchen Tools and Ingredients for Baby Food Preparation

The journey of preparing nutritious baby food is not just a culinary adventure but also a practical endeavor that requires the right tools and ingredients. Creating wholesome meals for your little one becomes a seamless and enjoyable process when you have the essential kitchen equipment and quality ingredients at your disposal.

Essential kitchen tools:

- **Blender or Food Processor**

A reliable blender or food processor is a cornerstone for preparing smooth purees and mashes. It ensures a consistent texture, making it easier for your baby to transition to solid foods.

- **Steamer Basket**

Steaming retains the maximum nutrients in fruits and vegetables. A steamer basket simplifies the process, allowing you to cook a variety of produce while preserving its natural goodness.

- **Mesh Strainer or Sieve**

For those early stages when you introduce solids, a mesh strainer or sieve helps remove any coarse bits, creating smoother purees suitable for your baby's developing palate.

- **Small Storage Containers**

Portion control is key. Invest in small, airtight storage containers to freeze and store individual servings of baby food. This makes meal preparation efficient and allows for easy portioning.

- **Baby Food Trays**

Specifically designed trays with small compartments are perfect for freezing and storing baby food in pre-portioned servings. This aids in organization and simplifies meal planning.

- **Soft Baby Spoons**

Soft, flexible spoons designed for baby feeding are gentle on your little one's gums and are the ideal utensil for introducing solids.

Quality Ingredients for Wholesome Baby Food:

- **Fresh Fruits and Vegetables**

Opt for a variety of fresh, seasonal fruits and vegetables. These provide essential vitamins, minerals, and fiber crucial for your baby's growth and development.

- **Whole Grains**

Introduce whole grains such as rice, oats, quinoa, and barley for added nutrients and fiber. These grains contribute to a well-rounded diet and support digestive health.

- **Lean Proteins**

Incorporate lean protein sources like chicken, turkey, lentils, and beans to provide the necessary building blocks for your baby's developing muscles and tissues.

- **Healthy Fats**

Include sources of healthy fats, such as avocados, olive oil, and nut butters. These fats are essential for brain development and overall growth.

- **Dairy or Dairy Alternatives**

Depending on your baby's age and dietary preferences, include dairy or fortified dairy alternatives for calcium and vitamin D, which are crucial for bone health.

- **Herbs and Spices**

As your baby grows, gradually introduce mild herbs and spices like cinnamon, basil, and mint to enhance flavors. These additions contribute to a diverse and enjoyable palate.

- **Iron-Rich Foods**

Ensure an adequate intake of iron through ingredients like fortified cereals, meats, and dark leafy greens. Iron is crucial for preventing anemia and supporting cognitive development.

- **Plain Yogurt or Probiotic-rich Foods**

Introduce plain yogurt or other probiotic-rich foods to promote a healthy gut microbiome. A well-balanced gut contributes to overall immune system function.

Planning Balanced Meals for Your Little One

That your baby receives a well-balanced diet is crucial for their overall growth, development, and long-term health. Planning nutritious and balanced meals involves considering various factors, including the right combination of food groups, portion sizes, and the introduction of diverse flavors and textures.

- **Understanding Nutritional Needs**

Begin by understanding your baby's nutritional needs at different stages of development. Factors such as age, weight, and activity level play a role in determining the appropriate balance of nutrients.

- **Incorporating a Variety of Food Groups**

Aim for a diverse range of food groups in each meal. Include fruits, vegetables, proteins, whole grains, and dairy or dairy alternatives to provide a broad spectrum of essential vitamins and minerals.

- **Gradual Introduction of Solids**

Introduce solids gradually, starting with single-ingredient purees and progressing to more complex blends. This approach allows your baby to adapt to new flavors and textures while ensuring they receive a variety of nutrients.

- **Portion Control and Frequency**

Pay attention to portion sizes suitable for your baby's age. Small, frequent meals throughout the day are often more manageable for little ones, helping to meet their energy and nutrient requirements.

- **Balancing Macronutrients**

Ensure a balance of macronutrients—carbohydrates, proteins, and fats. Carbohydrates provide energy, proteins support growth, and fats are essential for brain development. Adjusting the ratios based on your baby's age and developmental stage is key.

- **Age-Appropriate Texture Progression**

Progressively introduce a variety of textures as your baby grows. Starting with smooth purees, you can gradually transition to mashed foods, soft solids, and eventually finger foods. This progression supports oral motor development.

- **Customizing Meals to Preferences**

Pay attention to your baby's preferences and adapt meals accordingly. While introducing new foods, observe reactions and tailor future meals to include favorites while gently encouraging exploration of new tastes.

- **Considering Dietary Restrictions**

Be mindful of any dietary restrictions or allergies your baby may have. Consult with a pediatrician if you suspect allergies, and gradually introduce potential allergens one at a time, watching for any adverse reactions.

- **Hydration**

Include water in your baby's diet, especially as they start consuming solids. Proper hydration is essential for overall health, and offering sips of water between meals supports hydration without interfering with nutrient intake.

- **Creating a Routine**

Establishing a mealtime routine contributes to a sense of security for your baby. Consistent meal schedules help regulate hunger and foster a positive attitude towards food.

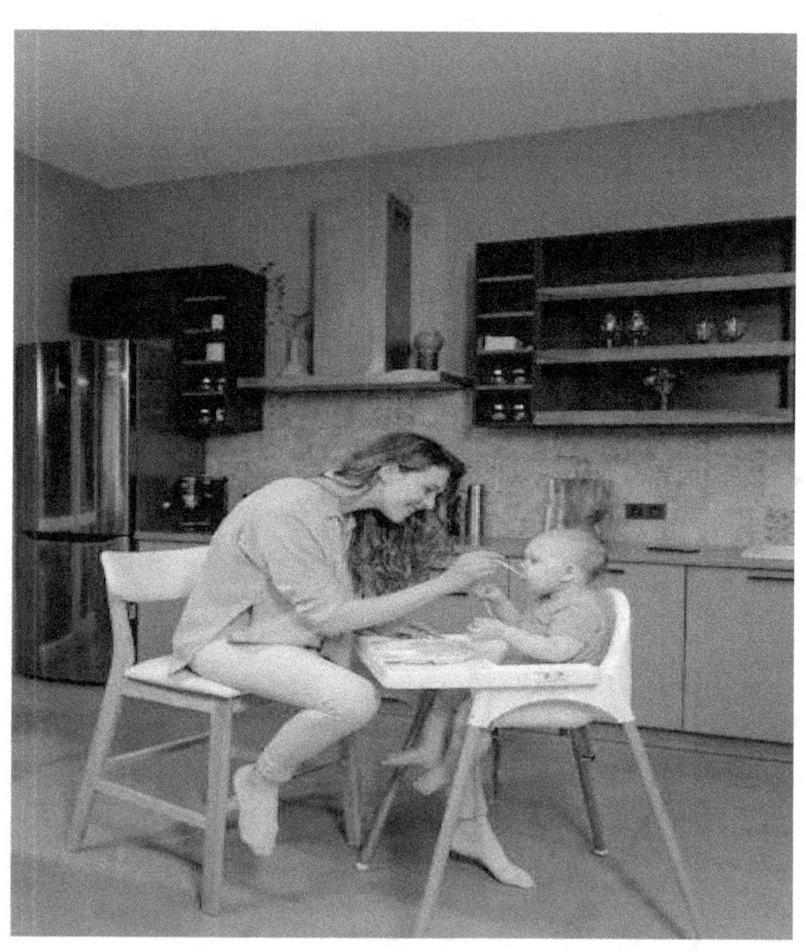

CHAPTER 2

First Bites: Introducing Solids

- **Transitioning from Milk to Solids**

The transition from exclusive milk feeding to the introduction of solid foods is a significant milestone in your baby's nutritional journey. This period marks a time of exploration, discovery, and the gradual development of new eating habits. Understanding the process and approaching it with patience and care is essential for a smooth and positive experience.

- **Recognizing Signs of Readiness**

Before starting the transition, observe your baby for signs of readiness. These may include the ability to sit with support, showing interest in watching others eat, and displaying increased tongue control.

- **Introducing Single-Ingredient Purees**

Begin the journey by introducing single-ingredient purees. These could include mild fruits like apples or pears or vegetables such as sweet potatoes or carrots. Single-ingredient foods help identify any potential allergies or sensitivities.

- **Gradual Progression to Mixed Textures**

As your baby becomes accustomed to purees, gradually progress to thicker textures and mixed combinations. This transition allows them to experience a variety of flavors and textures, aiding in the development of oral motor skills.

- **Timing and Frequency**

Start with one meal a day and gradually increase the frequency as your baby becomes more comfortable with solids. This gentle approach allows their digestive system to adapt to the new foods.

- **Offering a Variety of Nutrient-Rich Foods**

Provide a variety of nutrient-rich foods to ensure a well-rounded diet. Include fruits, vegetables, grains, and proteins, adjusting the texture and consistency based on your baby's developmental stage.

- **Encouraging Self-Feeding**

Introduce finger foods and encourage self-feeding as your baby's fine motor skills develop. This not only fosters independence but also enhances the sensory experience of mealtime.

- **Adapting to Preferences and Tastes**

Pay attention to your baby's preferences and adapt meals accordingly. While introducing a diverse range of foods, be flexible and cater to their evolving tastes to create a positive association with solids.

- **Maintaining Milk Feedings**

Remember that milk (breast milk or formula) continues to be an important part of your baby's diet during the transition to solids. Gradually, as solids become a more significant part of their diet, milk feedings can naturally adjust.

- **Watching for Allergic Reactions**

Be vigilant for any signs of allergic reactions when introducing new foods. Common allergens like eggs, dairy, and nuts can be introduced one at a time, with a few days in between, to monitor for any adverse responses.

- **Consultation with Pediatrician**

Always consult with your pediatrician before starting the transition to solids. They can provide guidance on appropriate foods and textures and ensure that your baby's nutritional needs are met during this crucial stage.

Age-appropriate foods for Your Baby

Introducing your baby to solid foods is a momentous occasion that requires thoughtful consideration of age-appropriate choices. The journey of discovering the right first foods is not only about nourishment but also about establishing positive eating habits. Here's a guide to help you navigate this exciting phase of your baby's nutritional development.

- **The Ideal Starting Age**

Begin introducing solid foods around the age of 6 months, as most babies have developed the necessary motor skills and digestive capacity. However, it's essential to observe your baby's individual signs of readiness.

- **Single-Ingredient Purees**

Start with single-ingredient purees to identify any potential allergies or sensitivities. Opt for mild and easily digestible options such as rice cereal, applesauce, or mashed banana.

- **Iron-Rich Foods**

Prioritize iron-rich foods like pureed meats, fortified cereals, and legumes. Iron is essential for the general and cognitive development of your child.

- **Vegetables and Fruits**

Introduce a variety of vegetables and fruits to provide a spectrum of vitamins and minerals. Begin with soft options like sweet potatoes, peas, avocados, and pears.

- **Gradual Texture Progression**

Gradually progress from smooth purees to slightly thicker textures as your baby becomes accustomed to swallowing. This progression supports the development of oral motor skills.

- **Introduction of Whole Grains**

Introduce whole grains like oatmeal, quinoa, and brown rice to provide fiber and additional nutrients. These grains contribute to a well-rounded diet and support digestive health.

- **Dairy or Dairy Alternatives**

Around 8–10 months, introduce small amounts of plain, full-fat yogurt or mashed cheese. These dairy sources offer calcium and healthy fats essential for bone and brain development.

- **Finger Foods and Self-Feeding**

Introduce age-appropriate finger foods like small pieces of soft fruits, cooked vegetables, or baby-friendly crackers. Encouraging self-feeding enhances fine motor skills and fosters independence.

- **Watch for Allergic Reactions**

Be vigilant for signs of allergies when introducing common allergens like eggs, dairy, and nuts. To avoid any negative reactions, introduce one new food at a time and wait a few days before introducing another.

- **Balanced Nutritional Variety**

Aim for a balanced variety of foods to ensure your baby receives a broad range of nutrients. The goal is to provide a diverse and nutritious diet that supports their growth and development.

- **Consistency and Patience**

Consistency is key during this phase. Continue offering a variety of foods and textures, and be patient as your baby explores and adapts to the world of solids.

- **Consultation with Pediatrician**

Always consult with your pediatrician before introducing new foods to ensure they align with your baby's individual needs and developmental milestones.

CHAPTER 3

Simple Fruit Blends for Your Baby's Palate

Introducing simple fruit blends is an exciting step in transitioning your baby to solid foods. These delightful combinations not only provide essential vitamins and minerals but also introduce a medley of flavors that can captivate your little one's taste buds. Here's a guide to creating simple and nutritious fruit blends for this special stage of your baby's culinary journey.

- **Starting with Single Fruits**

Begin by introducing single fruits to observe your baby's preferences and any potential reactions. Soft fruits like ripe bananas, mashed avocados, and pureed apples are gentle options for the initial stages.

- **Gradual Introduction of Variety**

Gradually expand the variety of fruits as your baby becomes more accustomed to solids. Include fruits with different textures and tastes, such as pears, peaches, and plums.

- **Creating Smooth Purees**

Create smooth purees by blending fruits with a bit of water or baby formula to achieve a consistency that is easy for your baby to swallow. Consistency is key in the early stages of introducing fruits.

- **Combining Complementary Flavors**

Explore combining complementary flavors to enhance the appeal of fruit blends. For example, pair sweet fruits like mango with a touch of creamy yogurt or mix apples with a hint of cinnamon for added warmth.

- **Introducing Berry Blends**

Berries are nutrient-packed and bring vibrant colors to your baby's plate. Introduce blueberries, strawberries, or raspberries after ensuring they are cut into small, manageable pieces or blended into a smooth consistency.

- **Adding Nutrient Boosters**

Consider adding nutrient boosters to your fruit blends, such as chia seeds for added fiber or a sprinkle of ground flaxseeds for omega-3 fatty acids. These additions contribute to the nutritional value of the blends.

- **Freeze for Teething Relief**

Freeze fruit blends into popsicle molds for a soothing and nutritious treat during teething. This not only provides relief but also introduces a novel and enjoyable way for your baby to experience flavors.

- **Textural Exploration**

As your baby progresses, introduce slightly chunkier textures. This can involve mashing softer fruits like ripe bananas with a fork, offering a textural transition to more complex fruit combinations.

- **Homemade Fruit Cups**

Create homemade fruit cups with a mix of diced fruits. This encourages self-feeding and adds a playful element to mealtime.

- **Monitoring for Allergies**

While introducing new fruits, monitor your baby for any signs of allergies or sensitivities. Proceed cautiously, introducing one fruit at a time and waiting a few days before introducing another.

- **Adjusting Consistency Over Time**

Adjust the consistency of fruit blends over time to align with your baby's developmental stage. Gradually transitioning from smooth purees to slightly chunkier textures supports oral motor development.

Exploring Vegetable Medleys for Tiny Taste Buds

Introducing vegetable medleys to your baby's diet is a wonderful way to expose them to a diverse range of flavors, textures, and essential nutrients. These colorful combinations not only provide a nutritional boost but also help develop a palate that appreciates the goodness of vegetables. Here's a guide to crafting delightful vegetable medleys for your little one's tiny taste buds.

- **Begin with Mild Vegetables**

Start by introducing mild and easily digestible vegetables to familiarize your baby with new flavors. Options like sweet potatoes, carrots, and peas are excellent choices for the initial stages.

- **Gradual Introduction of Variety**

Gradually expand the variety of vegetables in your baby's diet. Introduce different colors and textures, such as zucchini, butternut squash, and green beans, to create a medley of nutritional goodness.

- **Create Balanced Blends**

Craft well-balanced vegetable medleys by combining a mix of root vegetables, leafy greens, and cruciferous vegetables. This ensures a diverse array of vitamins, minerals, and antioxidants.

- **Steam or Roast for Retained Nutrients**

Steam or roast vegetables to retain their nutritional value. These cooking methods preserve the natural flavors and textures while maintaining the essential vitamins and minerals.

- **Incorporate Fresh Herbs**

Enhance the flavor profile of vegetable medleys by incorporating fresh herbs like parsley, dill, or cilantro. Herbs not only add a burst of freshness but also introduce your baby to a variety of tastes.

- **Texture Progression**

Progressively adjust the texture of vegetable medleys as your baby becomes more comfortable with solids. Start with finely pureed mixtures and gradually introduce slightly chunkier textures for oral motor development.

- **Introduction of Leafy Greens**

Introduce leafy greens like spinach or kale, ensuring they are finely chopped or cooked to a soft consistency. Leafy greens offer a rich source of iron and other essential nutrients.

- **Pairing Vegetables with Whole Grains**

Combine vegetable medleys with whole grains like quinoa or brown rice to create a more filling and nutritionally balanced meal. This introduces additional textures and flavors to your baby's palate.

- **Finger-Friendly Vegetable Options**

Introduce finger-friendly vegetable options like steamed broccoli florets or carrot sticks for self-feeding. Encouraging independent eating supports fine motor skills and fosters a sense of autonomy.

- **Colorful Presentation**

Present vegetable medleys in a visually appealing manner. Combining vibrant colors not only stimulates your baby's visual senses but also makes mealtime more enticing.

- **Adjusting Seasonings**

Gradually experiment with mild seasonings, such as a dash of mild spices or a hint of olive oil. Keep seasonings simple and age-appropriate while introducing your baby to a variety of flavors.

- **Monitoring for Allergies**

As with any new food introduction, monitor your baby for signs of allergies. Introduce one vegetable at a time and wait a few days before introducing another to observe any potential reactions.

Protein-Rich Purees for Growing Little Ones

Introducing protein-rich purees into your baby's diet is a significant step in providing essential nutrients crucial for their growth and development. These purees not only offer a diverse array of flavors but also ensure that your little one receives a balanced intake of proteins necessary for muscle development, immune function, and overall well-being. Here's a guide to crafting delightful and nutritious protein-rich purees for your growing baby.

- **Optimal Protein Sources**

Begin by selecting optimal protein sources suitable for your baby's age. Options such as pureed chicken, turkey, lentils, and beans provide essential amino acids necessary for their developing bodies.

- **Gradual Introduction of Proteins**

Gradually introduce protein-rich purees after your baby has experienced single-ingredient fruits and vegetables. This gradual progression allows their taste buds to adapt to new flavors while ensuring proper nutrition.

- **Creating Balanced Combinations**

Craft balanced, protein-rich purees by combining protein sources with mild vegetables or fruits. For example, blend chicken with sweet potatoes or lentils with carrots to create flavorful and nutritious blends.

- **Fortifying with Iron**

Many protein-rich foods, especially meats, are excellent sources of iron. Iron is vital for cognitive development and overall health. Incorporate iron-rich purees like pureed beef or lentil purees to support your baby's iron needs.

- **Cooking and Blending Techniques**

Opt for cooking methods that retain the nutritional value of proteins, such as steaming or boiling. Use a blender to achieve a smooth and easily digestible consistency, ensuring that the puree is suitable for your baby's developmental stage.

- **Introduction of Fish Purees**

Introduce fish purees rich in omega-3 fatty acids. Pureed salmon or mackerel provide essential nutrients for brain development. Ensure that the fish is cooked thoroughly and deboned before pureeing.

- **Plant-Based Protein Options**

Explore plant-based protein options such as pureed beans, chickpeas, or tofu for a vegetarian approach. These alternatives offer a variety of flavors and textures while providing essential protein.

- **Incorporating Quinoa or Millet**

Enhance protein-rich purees by incorporating grains like quinoa or millet. These grains not only contribute to protein content but also offer additional nutrients and a pleasant texture.

- **Age-Appropriate Texture Progression**

Gradually progress from smoother purees to slightly chunkier textures as your baby becomes more adept at handling solid foods. Adjust the texture based on their developmental stage.

- **Experimenting with Seasonings**

Experiment with mild seasonings to enhance the flavor of protein-rich purees. Consider incorporating gentle herbs like parsley or thyme for added taste without overwhelming their developing palate.

- **Finger-Friendly Proteins**

Introduce finger-friendly proteins as your baby progresses in their self-feeding journey. Small, soft pieces of cooked chicken or tofu allow for exploration and independence during mealtime.

- **Monitoring for Allergies**

As with any new food introduction, monitor your baby for signs of allergies when introducing protein-rich purees. Introduce one protein source at a time and wait a few days before introducing another to observe any potential reactions.

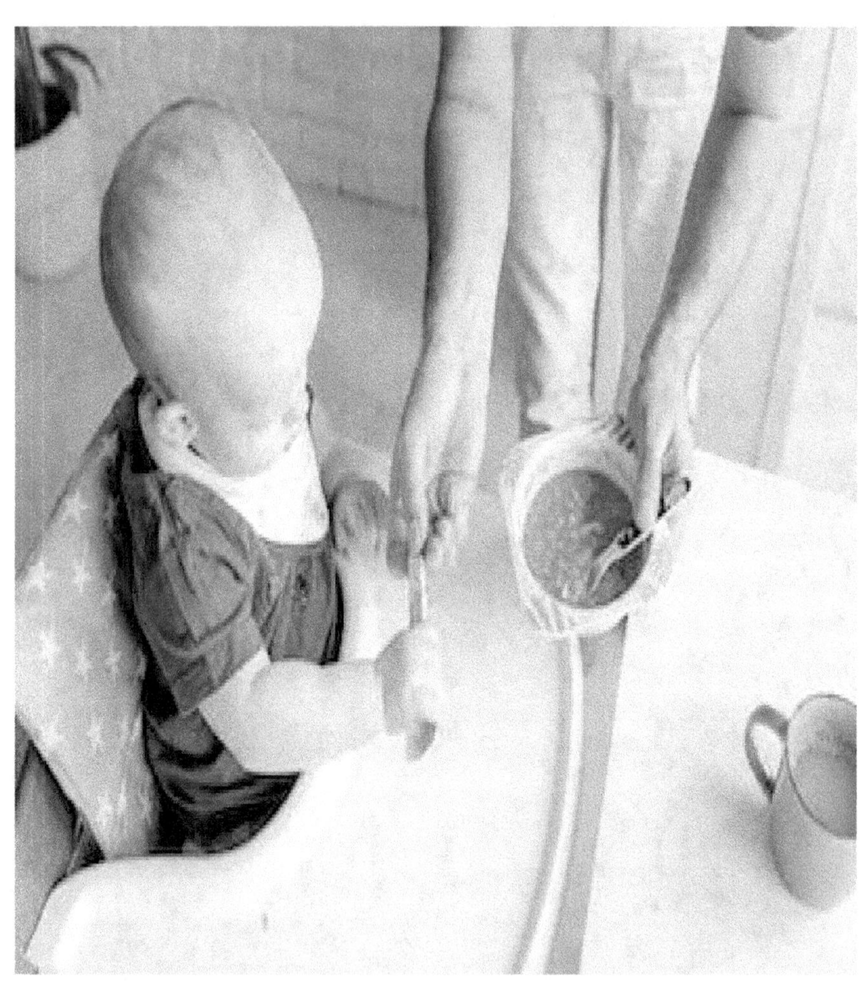

CHAPTER 4

Easy-to-Hold Snacks for Tiny Hands

As your baby progresses in their journey of self-feeding, introducing easy-to-hold snacks is a delightful way to encourage independence and fine motor skills. These snacks not only provide a source of nutrition but also allow your little one to explore different tastes and textures. Here's a guide to selecting and offering easy-to-hold snacks that are perfect for those tiny hands.

- **Optimal Snack Choices**

Choose snacks that are developmentally appropriate and easy for your baby to grasp. Options like soft fruits, steamed vegetables, or small pieces of cheese are excellent choices.

- **Bite-Sized Portions**

Offer snacks in bite-sized portions that are manageable for your baby. Cutting fruits or vegetables into small, easy-to-handle pieces reduces the risk of choking and promotes independent snacking.

- **Soft and Chewable Textures**

Opt for snacks with soft and chewable textures. This could include ripe banana slices, avocado chunks, or steamed sweet potato wedges that are gentle on your baby's emerging teeth.

- **Introducing Whole Grains**

Include whole-grain snacks like small pieces of lightly toasted bread, mini rice cakes, or puffed grains. These provide a source of carbohydrates and introduce different textures to your baby's palate.

- **Finger-Friendly Proteins**

Introduce finger-friendly proteins, such as small pieces of cooked chicken, tofu cubes, or shredded cheese. These snacks not only provide protein but also support your baby's growing muscles.

- **Fresh Fruit and Vegetable Sticks**

Offer fresh fruit or vegetable sticks that are easy to hold and nibble on. Carrot sticks, cucumber slices, or apple wedges are great options that allow for sensory exploration.

- **Yogurt Drops or Chilled Fruit Cubes**

Create yogurt drops or chilled fruit cubes by placing small portions on a tray and freezing them. These snacks not only soothe teething gums but also add a playful element to snack time.

- **Gradual Introduction of Nut Butters**

Gradually introduce nut butters by spreading a thin layer on small pieces of bread or offering nut butter on a baby-friendly cracker. Ensure the consistency is suitable for your baby's developmental stage.

- **Soft Cheese Cubes**

Offer soft cheese cubes that your baby can easily pick up. Cheeses like mild cheddar or mozzarella, cut into small pieces, provide both flavor and calcium.

- **Dried Fruit Bits**

Introduce dried fruit bits in small, bite-sized pieces. Make sure the dried fruits are soft and cut into appropriate sizes to avoid any choking hazards.

- **Monitoring for Allergies**

When introducing new snacks, be mindful of potential allergies. Introduce one new snack at a time and wait a few days before introducing another to monitor for any adverse reactions.

- **Supervised Self-Feeding**

Encourage supervised self-feeding during snack time. Allowing your baby to explore and interact with these easy-to-hold snacks fosters independence and builds confidence in their growing motor skills.

Soft Solids for Your Baby

The introduction to soft solids is a pivotal stage in your baby's culinary journey, marking the transition from purees to more textured foods. This exciting phase allows your little one to experience a variety of tastes, textures, and shapes, promoting oral motor development and independence. Here's a guide to navigating this stage with care and enthusiasm.

- **Signs of Readiness**

Look for signs of readiness in your baby, such as the ability to sit up with support, showing interest in your meals, and displaying improved tongue control. These signs indicate they might be ready for the transition to soft solids.

- **Start with Soft Purees**

Begin the journey by introducing soft purees with slightly thicker textures. Opt for purees with a chunkier consistency to acquaint your baby with the idea of varied textures in their meals.

- **Introduce Mashed and Minced Foods**

Progress to mashed and minced foods as your baby becomes more comfortable with textures. Soft-cooked vegetables, fruits, and well-cooked grains are excellent choices to promote chewing and swallowing.

- **Explore Different Textures**

Offer a diverse range of textures to enhance sensory exploration. Soft solids can include finely diced fruits, tender-cooked pasta, and minced meats, providing a variety of tactile experiences.

- **Finger Foods and Self-Feeding**

Introduce finger foods that are easy for your baby to grasp. Soft finger foods like small pieces of banana, cooked peas, or diced cheese encourage self-feeding, enhancing fine motor skills.

- **Gradual Introduction of Proteins**

Incorporate soft protein sources such as finely shredded chicken, flaked fish, or mashed beans. These additions provide essential nutrients for your baby's growth and development.

- **Cooked Grains and Cereals**

Introduce cooked grains like rice, quinoa, or oatmeal to expand the variety of textures in your baby's diet. Soft cereals are excellent options for introducing different grains.

- **Soft-cooked vegetables**

Offer soft-cooked vegetables like sweet potatoes, carrots, or peas in small, bite-sized pieces. Steaming or boiling vegetables until they are tender ensures they are easily mashable for your baby.

- **Monitor for Choking Hazards**

Be mindful of potential choking hazards. Cut foods into appropriate sizes, avoiding small, hard pieces that could pose a risk. Always supervise your baby during mealtime.

- **Experiment with Flavors**

Experiment with introducing different flavors to your baby. Add gentle herbs and spices to enhance the taste of soft solids, making mealtimes more enjoyable.

- **Gradual Transition to Family Foods**

Gradually transition your baby to family foods as they grow more accustomed to different textures. Continue to offer a mix of soft solids and gradually introduce foods with more complex textures.

- **Consultation with Pediatrician**

Keep open communication with your pediatrician throughout this process. They can offer guidance, ensure your baby's nutritional needs are met, and address any concerns you may have.

CHAPTER 5

Common Allergens for Your Baby

Introducing common allergens to your baby's diet is an important step in promoting tolerance and preventing allergies later in life. However, it requires careful consideration and a systematic approach to ensure your baby's safety. Here's a guide on how to safely introduce common allergens to your little one.

- **Consult with Your Pediatrician**

Before introducing any common allergens, consult with your pediatrician. They can provide personalized advice based on your baby's health history and individual risk factors.

- **Begin with Single Ingredients**

Start by introducing common allergens as single ingredients. For example, introduce pureed peanuts or peanut butter without combining them with other new foods. This approach helps pinpoint specific allergens if a reaction occurs.

- **Gradual Introduction**

Introduce one common allergen at a time, waiting several days before introducing another. This spacing allows you to monitor your baby for any potential allergic reactions.

- **Observe for Reactions**

Pay close attention to any signs of allergic reactions after introducing a new allergen. Common symptoms include hives, redness, swelling, vomiting, diarrhea, or difficulty breathing. If you observe any of these, seek immediate medical attention.

- **Timing of Introduction**

Introduce common allergens when your baby is developmentally ready, usually around 6 months of age. At this stage, their immune system is more mature, and they may be less likely to develop allergies.

- **Common Allergens to Introduce**

Consider introducing common allergens such as peanuts, tree nuts, eggs, milk, soy, wheat, fish, and shellfish. These foods provide essential nutrients and contribute to a well-rounded diet.

- **Peanut Allergen Introduction**

For peanuts, start with a small amount of smooth peanut butter or a peanut-containing food. Avoid whole peanuts, as they pose a choking hazard for babies.

- **Gradual Increase in Amounts**

If your baby tolerates the initial introduction of a common allergen, gradually increase the amounts over time. This progression helps build tolerance while minimizing the risk of adverse reactions.

- **Maintaining Regular Exposure**

Once common allergens are successfully introduced, maintain regular exposure to them in your baby's diet. Consistency can contribute to continued tolerance.

- **Allergen Introduction During Daytime**

Introduce common allergens during the day when medical assistance is more readily available. Avoid introducing new foods close to bedtime to ensure you can monitor your baby for reactions.

- **Allergen Introduction at Home**

Introduce common allergens at home rather than in public places or restaurants. This controlled environment allows for a prompt response if an allergic reaction occurs.

- **Gradual Introduction to Family Foods**

Gradually incorporate common allergens into family meals as your baby progresses to eating a wider variety of foods. This helps normalize these foods in their diet.

Monitoring for Allergic Reactions in Your Baby

As you introduce new foods to your baby's diet, vigilant monitoring for allergic reactions is crucial for their well-being. Being aware of potential signs and acting promptly ensures a safe and positive feeding experience. Here's a guide on how to monitor for allergic reactions and respond effectively.

- **Start with Single Ingredients**

Begin by introducing single ingredients to identify specific allergens. This approach helps pinpoint the cause of any potential reactions.

- **Observe Facial Changes**

Watch for facial changes, including redness, swelling, or hives around the mouth, eyes, or cheeks. These symptoms may be an indication of an allergic reaction.

- **Monitor for Gastrointestinal Symptoms**

Pay attention to gastrointestinal symptoms such as vomiting, diarrhea, or stomach discomfort. These can be indicators of an adverse reaction to a new food.

- **Respiratory Symptoms**

Be alert to respiratory symptoms such as coughing, wheezing, or difficulty breathing. These signs may suggest an allergic response affecting the respiratory system.

- **Watch for Behavioral Changes**

Observe any changes in your baby's behavior, such as irritability, fussiness, or lethargy. Unusual behavior may be a subtle sign of discomfort.

- **Be Mindful of Skin Reactions**

Check for skin reactions, including redness, itching, or the appearance of rashes. These symptoms may occur in various parts of the body.

- **Immediate Reactions**

Some allergic reactions can be immediate. If you notice symptoms within a short time after introducing a new food, seek prompt medical attention.

- **Delayed Reactions**

Some reactions may occur hours, or even days, after exposure to an allergen. Remain vigilant for delayed symptoms and consult with your pediatrician if you suspect an association with a specific food.

- **Documenting Food Introductions**

Keep a record of the foods introduced and any observed reactions. This documentation helps in identifying patterns and provides valuable information for healthcare professionals.

- **Emergency Response Plan**

Familiarize yourself with emergency response plans in case of severe allergic reactions (anaphylaxis). Know how to administer any prescribed medications and seek immediate medical help if needed.

Remember: Every baby is unique, and reactions to new foods can vary. If you suspect an allergic reaction, consult with your pediatrician promptly. Taking a cautious and informed approach to monitoring for allergic reactions ensures that your baby's introduction to solid foods is a safe and positive experience.

CHAPTER 6

Meal Ideas for Your Little Explorer

Making mealtimes a joyous adventure for your baby involves not only nourishing their growing bodies but also stimulating their curious minds. Here are creative and engaging meal ideas to turn each bite into an exploration, fostering a positive relationship with food for your little one.

- **Colorful Veggie Rainbow Plate**

Create a vibrant plate using a variety of colorful vegetables. Arrange diced red peppers, orange carrots, yellow squash, green peas, and purple cabbage in a rainbow formation. This not only provides a visual feast but also introduces different textures and flavors.

- **Shape-Shifting Sandwiches**

Transform sandwiches into exciting shapes using cookie cutters. Delight your baby with star-shaped peanut butter and banana sandwiches or heart-shaped cheese and cucumber bites.

- **Food Art on a Plate**

Turn the plate into a canvas by arranging food into fun shapes and characters. Use broccoli trees, carrot sticks as sunbeams, and mashed potato clouds to create a playful food landscape.

- **Mini Fruit Kebabs**

Thread bite-sized fruit pieces onto small skewers to create mini fruit kebabs. This not only adds a visual appeal but also encourages hand-eye coordination as your baby explores different fruits.

- **Mix-and-Match Tasting Platter**

Introduce a mix-and-match tasting platter with an assortment of small portions of fruits, vegetables, cheeses, and crackers. This allows your baby to explore various textures and flavors in a single meal.

- **Alphabet Pasta Adventure**

Incorporate alphabet-shaped pasta into meals for a playful learning experience. Spell out simple words or your baby's name on the plate to make mealtime an educational adventure.

- **Storybook-Inspired Meals**

Draw inspiration from your baby's favorite storybooks by creating meals based on characters or themes. Turn a bowl of oatmeal into a bear's porridge or shape pancakes into characters from beloved tales.

- **Dips and Dunking Fun**

Provide small bowls of nutritious dips like yogurt, hummus, or guacamole alongside bite-sized veggies or fruit slices. Encourage dipping and dunking for an interactive and enjoyable meal.

- **Food Puzzles and Shapes**

Cut foods into puzzle-like shapes or use cookie cutters to create interesting forms. Let your baby explore assembling the pieces, making mealtime a playful puzzle-solving experience.

- **Edible Finger Paints**

Create edible finger paints using yogurt dyed with natural food colors. Allow your baby to express their creativity by finger painting on a high-chair tray with these tasty and colorful paints.

- **DIY Snack Stations**

Set up DIY snack stations with a variety of healthy options. Let your baby explore and assemble their own snacks, fostering independence and decision-making skills.

- **Musical Food Play**

Introduce musical elements by tapping utensils on different food surfaces to create sounds. Turn mealtime into a sensory-rich experience that engages both taste and hearing.

Making Mealtime Enjoyable for Your Baby

Turning mealtime into an enjoyable experience for your baby goes beyond mere nutrition—it's about fostering positive associations with food and building a foundation for a lifetime of healthy eating habits. Here are strategies to make mealtime a joyful occasion for your little one:

- **Establish Routine and Consistency**

Set a regular mealtime routine to create a sense of predictability. Consistency helps your baby anticipate meals, making the dining experience more comfortable and enjoyable.

- **Create a Positive Atmosphere**

Foster a positive environment by maintaining a calm and cheerful atmosphere during meals. Positive feelings throughout mealtimes increase the likelihood that your baby will identify them with happiness.

- **Engaging Conversation**

Engage your baby in simple conversation during meals. Describe the colors, textures, and flavors of the food. This not only stimulates language development but also makes mealtime more interactive.

- **Offer Age-Appropriate Utensils**

Introduce age-appropriate utensils that are easy for your baby to handle. Child-friendly utensils make the dining experience more manageable and encourage self-feeding.

- **Playful Plating**

Present meals in a playful and visually appealing manner. Use colorful plates, arrange foods into fun shapes, or create food art to captivate your baby's interest.

- **Variety and Exploration**

Introduce a variety of foods to encourage exploration. Rotate different fruits, vegetables, and proteins to expose your baby to diverse tastes and textures.

- **Encourage Self-Feeding**

Gradually encourage self-feeding by offering bite-sized and easy-to-handle foods. Allowing your baby to explore and eat independently enhances their fine motor skills and fosters a sense of autonomy.

- **Introduce Novelty**

Introduce novelty by offering new foods or variations of familiar ones. This keeps mealtimes exciting and allows your baby to experience a broad spectrum of flavors.

- **Incorporate Fun Elements**

Incorporate fun elements like themed meals or incorporating favorite characters into the dining experience. Making mealtimes entertaining contributes to a positive attitude towards food.

- **Musical Accompaniment**

Play soft and soothing music during meals. Music can create a pleasant atmosphere, making mealtimes a more enjoyable and relaxed experience.

- **Celebrate Achievements**

Celebrate small milestones during meals. Whether it's trying a new food or successfully using a spoon, acknowledging achievements positively reinforces the dining experience.

- **Limit Distractions**

Minimize distractions during meals by creating a dedicated eating space. This helps your baby focus on the food and the sensory experience of eating.

- **Be Patient and Responsive**

Approach mealtime with patience. Let your infant explore and communicate what they want. Be responsive to their cues, recognizing when they are full or have particular preferences.

- **Role Modeling**

Be a positive role model by demonstrating healthy eating habits. Your baby is more likely to mimic your behavior and develop a positive attitude towards a variety of foods.

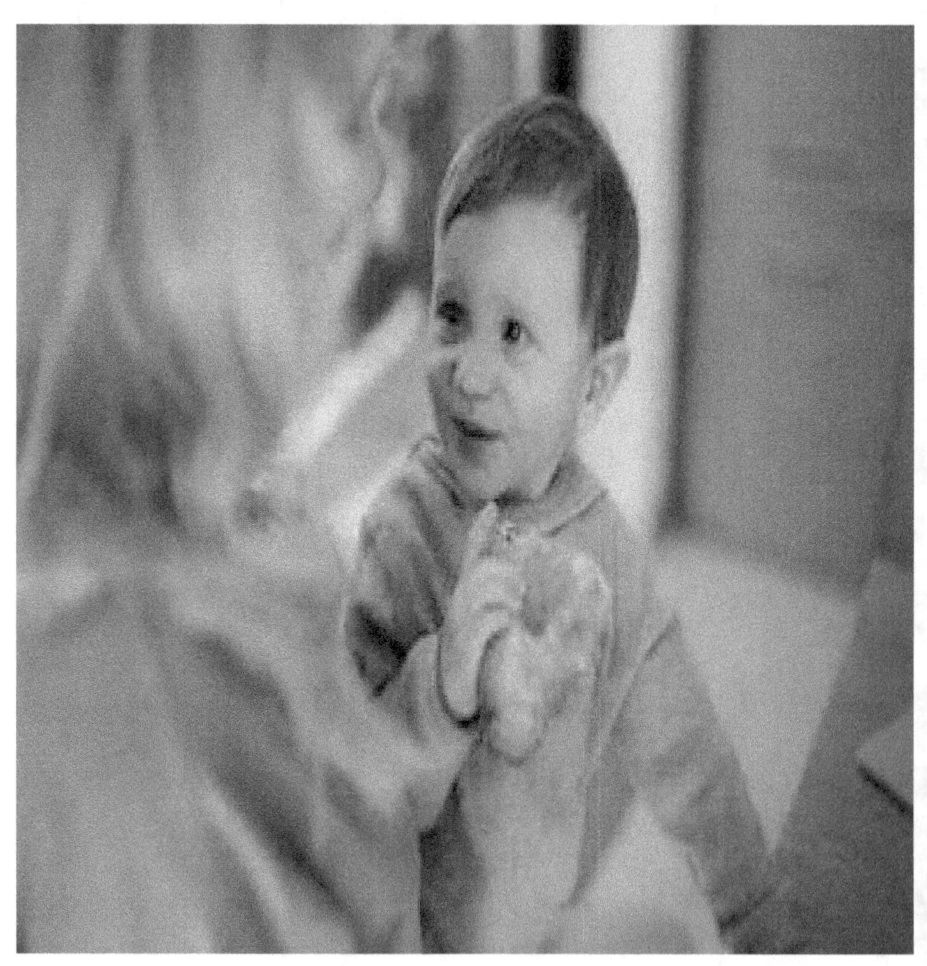

CHAPTER 7

Nutritional Tips for New Moms

Nurturing Your Baby's Health with a Well-Rounded Diet

Ensuring your baby receives a balanced diet is essential for their growth, development, and overall well-being. Crafting a diverse and nutrient-rich menu helps lay the foundation for healthy eating habits. Here's a comprehensive guide on how to maintain a balanced diet for your little one:

- **Foundation of Breast Milk or Formula**

Up to six months, breast milk or formula is the primary source of nutrition. Ensure your baby receives the recommended amount to support their growth and development.

- **Introduction of Solids**

Begin introducing solids around six months, starting with single-ingredient purees. Gradually progress to more textured foods as your baby develops the ability to chew and swallow.

- **The Four Main Food Groups**

Incorporate foods from the four main food groups: **fruits, vegetables, grains**, and **proteins**. This ensures a diverse array of nutrients essential for different aspects of your baby's development.

- **Fruit and Vegetable Rainbow**

Offer a colorful assortment of fruits and vegetables. Different colors represent various vitamins and minerals, contributing to your baby's overall health. Aim for variety to cover a broad nutritional spectrum.

- **Whole Grains for Energy**

Introduce whole grains such as brown rice, oats, and whole wheat. These provide essential carbohydrates for energy and fiber for digestive health.

- **Protein Power**

Include protein sources like lean meats, poultry, fish, eggs, dairy, legumes, and tofu. Proteins are crucial for muscle development, immune function, and overall growth.

- **Healthy Fats**

Incorporate healthy fats into your baby's diet. Avocado, nut butters, and olive oil are excellent sources of essential fats important for brain development.

- **Dairy for Calcium**

Include age-appropriate dairy or dairy alternatives to meet calcium needs for bone development. Options like yogurt and cheese provide additional textures and flavors.

- **Iron-Rich Foods**

Introduce iron-rich foods such as lean meats, fortified cereals, beans, and lentils. Iron is vital for cognitive development and overall health.

- **Hydration**

Offer water in a sippy cup once your baby starts eating solids. Hydration is crucial for overall well-being and supports digestion.

- **Limit Added Sugars and Salt**

Minimize the introduction of added sugars and salt. This helps cultivate a preference for natural flavors and reduces the risk of developing unhealthy eating habits.

- **Monitor Portion Sizes**

Be mindful of portion sizes suitable for your baby's age and developmental stage. Pay attention to the cues of hunger and fullness.

- **Gradual Introduction of Allergens**

Gradually introduce common allergens such as peanuts, tree nuts, eggs, and fish. Monitor for any adverse reactions and consult with your pediatrician if needed.

- **Regular Pediatric Checkups**

Schedule regular pediatric checkups to monitor your baby's growth, nutritional needs, and developmental milestones. Seek guidance from your healthcare provider on any dietary concerns.

- **Responsive Feeding**

Practice responsive feeding by recognizing and respecting your baby's hunger and fullness cues. This helps establish a healthy relationship with food.

A Guide to Self-Care for Mothers

Embarking on the journey of motherhood is a rewarding yet demanding experience, making self-care an essential component for the well-being of both you and your baby. Here's a guide on how to incorporate self-care practices into your routine to nurture yourself and, in turn, enhance your ability to care for your little one.

- **Prioritize Sleep**

Quality sleep is the cornerstone of self-care. Create a bedtime routine, take naps when possible, and enlist support from partners or family members to ensure you get the rest you need.

- **Nourishing Nutrition**

Maintain a balanced diet rich in nutrients. Nourishing your body with wholesome foods provides the energy and vitality needed to navigate the demands of motherhood.

- **Hydration Habits**

Stay hydrated throughout the day. Proper hydration supports overall health and energy levels and helps with postpartum recovery.

- **Exercise for Well-being**

Incorporate gentle exercises into your routine, tailored to your postpartum recovery. Activities like walking, yoga, or postnatal exercises can contribute to both physical and mental well-being.

- **Restorative Moments**

Carve out moments for self-reflection and relaxation. Whether it's a few quiet minutes with a cup of tea, deep breathing exercises, or mindfulness practices, these moments contribute to your emotional well-being.

- **Delegate and Accept Help**

Delegate tasks and accept help from loved ones. Whether it's assistance with household chores or someone watching the baby for a short period of time, sharing responsibilities lightens the load and allows you time for self-care.

- **Connection with Others**

Foster connections with friends and family. Social support is crucial for emotional well-being, providing an outlet to share experiences and receive encouragement.

- **Set Realistic Expectations**

Establish realistic expectations for yourself. Understand that it's okay not to be perfect, and each day may bring new challenges. Embrace flexibility and prioritize what truly matters.

- **Schedule "Me" Time**

Schedule dedicated "me" time regularly. Whether it's a solo walk, a hobby you enjoy, or even a quiet bath, these moments are essential for recharging your mental and emotional reserves.

- **Communication with Partner**

Maintain open communication with your partner. Share your needs and feelings, and collaborate on strategies to ensure both of you have time for self-care.

- **Professional Support**

Seek professional support if needed. Whether it's through counseling, therapy, or talking to a healthcare provider, reaching out for assistance is a courageous step toward self-care.

- **Positive Affirmations**

Practice positive affirmations. Remind yourself of your strength and capability as a mother. Cultivating a positive mindset contributes to overall well-being.

- **Engage in Hobbies**

Engage in hobbies or activities you enjoy. Whether it's reading, crafting, or pursuing a creative outlet, investing time in your passions enhances your sense of self.

- **Celebrate Achievements**

Celebrate and give thanks for all of your accomplishments, large and small. Recognizing your efforts fosters a sense of accomplishment and self-worth.

- **Regular Health Check-ups**

Prioritize regular health check-ups for yourself. Monitoring your physical and mental health ensures you can address any concerns proactively.

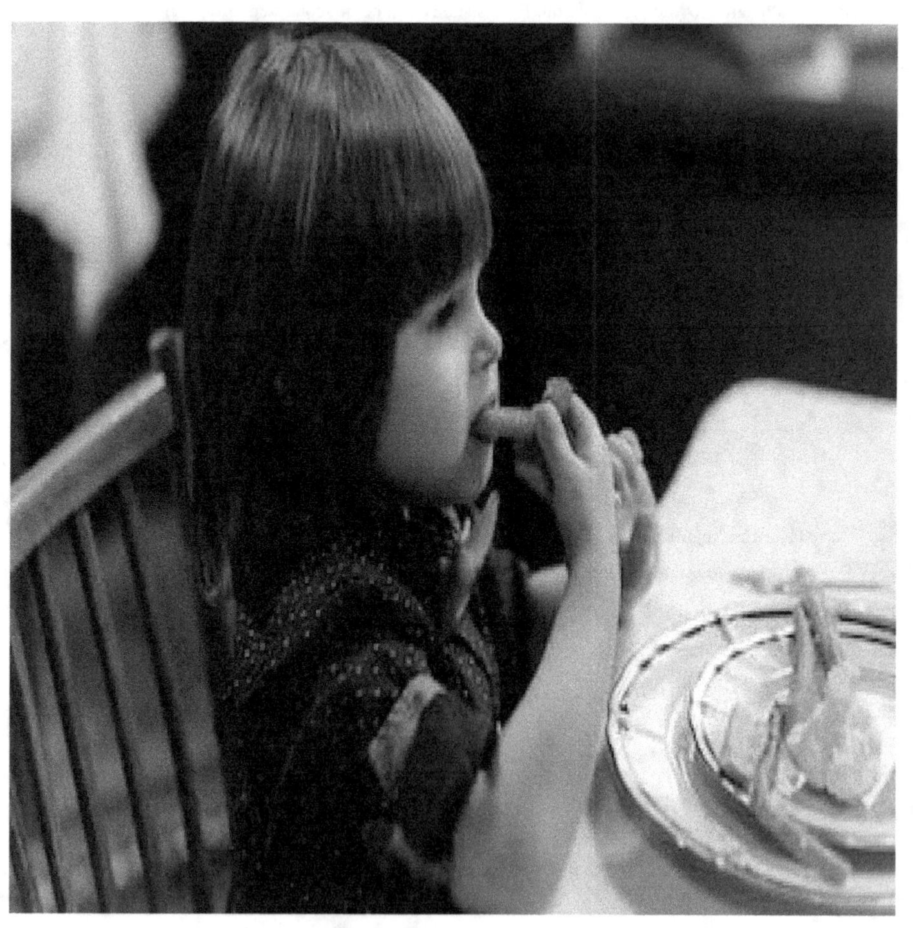

CHAPTER 8

Addressing Common Concerns with Confidence

The journey of motherhood comes with its share of joys and challenges. Addressing common concerns is a natural part of this transformative experience. Here's a guide to help you navigate through some typical worries and uncertainties, empowering you with the confidence to embrace and overcome them.

- **Sleep Deprivation**

Concern: Lack of sleep is a common worry for new mothers. Sleepless nights can leave you feeling exhausted and overwhelmed.

Solution: Establish a consistent bedtime routine, take short naps when the baby sleeps, and consider sharing nighttime responsibilities with your partner or a trusted family member.

- **Postpartum Body Changes**

Concern: Changes in your body postpartum can be challenging, affecting self-esteem and body image.

Solution: Embrace self-love and self-acceptance. Focus on your body's incredible ability to nurture life. Engage in gentle exercises, and prioritize nourishing your body with healthy foods.

- **Balancing Work and Motherhood**

Concern: Balancing a career with motherhood can be a source of stress and guilt.

Solution: Establish clear boundaries, communicate openly with your employer about flexible work arrangements, and build a support network. Always keep in mind that asking for assistance is OK.

- **Feeding Challenges**

Concern: Breastfeeding or formula feeding challenges can be emotionally and physically taxing.

Solution: Seek guidance from lactation consultants or healthcare professionals. If formula feeding, choose a formula that meets your baby's nutritional needs. Remember that feeding is best, and prioritize what works best for you and your baby.

- **Postpartum Depression**

Concern: Mothers may experience postpartum depression, which is a genuine and widespread fear.

Solution: Seek support from healthcare professionals, family, and friends. Open communication about your feelings is crucial. Always keep in mind that asking for assistance does not indicate weakness but rather strength.

- **Developmental Milestone**

Concern: Worrying about your baby's developmental milestones is normal, especially for first-time mothers.

Solution: Trust the process and appreciate that every baby develops at their own pace. Regular pediatric check-ups can provide reassurance, and consulting with healthcare providers can address specific concerns.

- **Mom Guilt**

Concern: Feeling guilty about taking time for yourself or making certain parenting choices is a common struggle.

Solution: Acknowledge that self-care is crucial for your well-being and your ability to care for your baby. Trust your instincts, and remember that there is no one-size-fits-all approach to parenting.

- **Relationship Changes**

Concern: Adjusting to changes in your relationship with your partner after having a baby can be challenging.

Solution: Prioritize open communication, express your needs, and make time for each other. Understanding that relationships evolve and finding new ways to connect is essential.

- **Time Management**

Concern: Juggling multiple responsibilities and managing time effectively can be overwhelming.

Solution: Prioritize tasks, delegate when possible, and don't hesitate to ask for help. Creating a realistic schedule can help manage expectations and reduce stress.

- **Comparison to Others**

Concern: Comparing yourself to other mothers or societal expectations can lead to feelings of inadequacy.

Solution: Focus on your unique journey and your baby's individual needs. Every mother has her own set of challenges and strengths. Seek support from other mothers who provide understanding and encouragement.

- **Isolation as a Mother**

Concern: How Do I Deal with Feelings of Isolation as a New Mother?

Solution: Cultivate a support network, engage with other mothers, and join parenting groups. Participate in community activities and be open to making new connections.

- **Prioritize self-care.**

Concern: How Can I Prioritize Self-Care in My Busy Schedule?

Solution: Schedule dedicated "me" time regularly. Whether it's a solo walk, a hobby you enjoy, or even a quiet bath, these moments are essential for recharging your mental and emotional reserves.

CONCLUSION

Celebrating Milestones

As your little one embarks on the culinary journey, each spoonful becomes a milestone, marking significant developmental stages. Celebrate these moments with joy and enthusiasm, turning feeding time into a delightful exploration. Here's a guide to celebrating your baby's culinary milestones:

- **First Taste Adventures**

Celebrate the introduction of your baby's first tastes with excitement and encouragement. Capture their adorable expressions as they experience new flavors and textures.

- **Successful Spoon Feeding**

Rejoice when your baby starts mastering the art of spoon-feeding. This milestone marks the beginning of their ability to self-feed and develop fine motor skills.

- **Transition to Solid Foods**

Celebrate the transition from purees to solid foods. Offer a variety of textures, allowing your baby to explore and enjoy the sensory experience of different consistencies.

- **Independent Finger Foods**

Applaud the moment your baby starts picking up and feeding themselves with finger foods. This newfound independence is a significant step in their self-feeding journey.

- **Variety of Tastes and Flavors**

Introduce a diverse range of tastes and flavors to your baby's palate. Celebrate the acceptance of various fruits, vegetables, and proteins, fostering a love for a variety of nutritious foods.

- **First Attempts at Drinking from a Cup**

Mark the occasion when your baby takes their first sips from a cup. Whether using a sippy cup or an open cup, this milestone signifies growing coordination and independence.

- **Exploring New Cuisines**

Introduce your baby to different cuisines from around the world. Celebrate the joy of discovering diverse flavors, spices, and cultural dishes together.

- **Family Mealtime Traditions**

Embrace family mealtime traditions as your baby becomes an active participant. Whether it's a special recipe passed down through generations or a weekly family dinner, these traditions create lasting memories.

- **Transition to a Variety of Textures**

Celebrate the successful transition to a wide range of textures, including soft solids, mashed foods, and chunkier options. This milestone contributes to the development of chewing skills.

- **Gradual Introduction to Family Foods**

Rejoice as your baby gradually integrates into family meals. Celebrate the inclusivity of shared meals and the joy of watching your little one enjoy the same foods as the rest of the family.

- **First Attempt at Self-Feeding with Utensils**

Applaud your baby's first attempts at self-feeding with utensils. This milestone signals growing independence and improved hand-eye coordination.

- **Developing Food Preferences**

Recognize and celebrate your baby's developing food preferences. As they express likes and dislikes, tailor meals to incorporate their favored ingredients while still introducing new ones.

- **Transition to Three Meals a Day**

Celebrate the transition to three meals a day as your baby's nutritional needs evolve. This milestone signifies their increasing capacity for a more structured eating routine.

Family Celebrations and Special Occasions

Make family celebrations and special occasions a culinary adventure. Whether it's a birthday cake or a holiday feast, these moments create cherished memories around food.

- **Gradual Transition to Adult Foods**

Celebrate the gradual transition to adult foods. As your baby's taste buds evolve, embrace the joy of sharing meals that cater to their growing preferences.

THE CONCLUSION

As we draw the curtain on the pages of "Nourishing Start: Easy and Tasty Baby Food Ideas for New Mothers," we extend heartfelt congratulations on embarking on this culinary journey with your precious little one. This book has been crafted not just as a guide but as a companion, sharing in the joy, challenges, and triumphs of nurturing your baby through the magical world of food.

In these pages, you've explored expert-backed advice, nutrient-rich recipes, and practical tips aimed at transforming mealtimes into moments of connection and nourishment. As your baby transitions from the first tastes of purees to the exciting adventures of self-feeding, we hope you've discovered the joy of crafting meals that go beyond sustenance, becoming a source of love, exploration, and shared delight.

Key Takeaways

Knowledge Empowerment: The journey of motherhood comes with a myriad of questions, and "Nourishing Start" aims to provide not just answers but a foundation of knowledge. Empowered with insights into your baby's nutritional needs, you're now equipped to make informed choices that contribute to their health and well-being.

Culinary Creativity: Your kitchen has transformed into a playground of creativity, where each ingredient is carefully chosen to delight your baby's developing palate. Whether it's the first taste of a new flavor or the introduction of diverse textures, you've embraced the art of culinary creation.

Positive Mealtime Atmosphere: Mealtime is no longer just a routine; it's a cherished moment of connection. Through the guidance in this book, you've fostered a positive atmosphere, turning mealtimes into enjoyable experiences that not only nourish the body but also nurture the bond between you and your little one.

Building Healthy Habits: The foundation for a lifetime of healthy eating habits has been laid. By introducing a variety of nutrient-rich foods, navigating developmental milestones, and encouraging self-feeding, you've played a pivotal role in shaping your baby's relationship with food for years to come.

Celebrating Milestones: Alongside the recipes and tips, you've celebrated countless milestones, from the first taste to the triumphant moments of self-feeding. Each page turned in this book marked a step forward in your baby's culinary journey, and we trust that these milestones will be etched in your heart forever.

Looking Forward:

As you close this book, remember that the adventure doesn't end here. It continues in the giggles shared over a messy high chair, in the exploration of new flavors, and in the delightful moments of discovering your baby's unique food preferences. Continue to savor these precious times, adapting the knowledge and skills gained from "Nourishing Start" to the evolving stages of your baby's growth.

May your kitchen always be filled with the aroma of love, and may each spoonful be a testament to the care and dedication you invest in your baby's well-being. I wish you and your little one a continued journey of delightful discoveries and nourishment that goes beyond the plate.

We appreciate your willingness to include "Nourishing Start" in your narrative. Happy feeding, happy bonding, and here's to a future filled with many more delicious moments with your little one.